Negative Calorie Diet

Cookbook & Guide Which Will Help You To Burn Body Fat, Lose Weight And Live Healthy

LELA GIBSON

CONTENTS

LELA GIBSON

Introduction

I would like to thank you for buying the book, "Negative Calorie Diet".

This book contains proven steps and strategies on how to burn body fat, lose weight and eat healthy.

Are you on the verge of giving up on your weight loss goals? Have you tried reducing your fat intake, eating fewer carbohydrates and all the diets that call for eating fewer proteins and carbohydrates, drank a lot of water, but you don't lose any weight? Does nothing seem to work? Well, I guess losing hope is understandable, but wait, DO NOT GIVE UP JUST YET! There is one more option, the best option in fact: The Negative Calorie Diet.

If we are to go by the facts, the Negative Calorie Diet is the fastest way to lose weight; you can lose up to 14 pounds a week when you adopt the diet! Thanks to this diet, losing weight is no longer a random dream or a hope; it is a reality for thousands of people across the globe.

In this book, you will learn more about the negative calorie diet, how it works and some amazing recipes that will help you burn fat.

Be sure to like us on Facebook.

Thanks again for buying this book, I hope you enjoy it!

LELA GIBSON

Negative Calorie Diet: What Is It

This unique diet draws upon the idea that some foods have the 'negative calorie' effect that we ought to consider in burning fat. A food is considered to have a negative calorie effect when the calories these foods use to digest are typically higher than the calories in the foods themselves.

When you eat something, you begin by chewing, a process that consumes energy. Some foods such as those higher in stringy fibers like celery will require more chewing, which will result in more energy expenditure, and there are others like pasta and cakes that don't require as much chewing.

After chewing, the foods go to the stomach through the esophagus and the other processes of digestion take over until absorption takes place and the body excretes the residual mass.

With negative calorie foods, this entire process uses up more calories than the foods have. The extra calories the body has to provide in order to process the foods are taken from the fat stores, and the more of these negative calorie foods you eat, the more your fat stores will lose calories, and as a result, the more fat you will lose.

Let us take broccoli as an example: 100 grams (contains 25 calories).

When you eat 100 grams of broccoli, it takes your body about 80 calories worth of energy to digest it. This results in a net calorie use of 55 calories that should come from the fat stores in your body. As you can see, the 55 calories make up the negative net calorie.

Let us now take a counter example of a piece of cake containing 400 calories.

Your body will take about 150 calories to digest the piece of cake, leaving net 250 calories deposited in the body and stored as fat.

The negative calorie diet consists of over 100 foods proven to have negative calorie qualities. Most of these foods are fruits and veggies that are high in fiber. Let us look at them in more detail in the following chapter.

Negative Calorie Food List

Here is a list of negative calorie foods:

Vegetables

As you already know, fibrous, complex carbohydrates epitomize the negative calorie diet. The American Heart Association actually recommends that we strive to get more than half of our daily calories from complex carbohydrates. Furthermore, consuming the correct amounts of fiber is great for your digestive process since it helps your body eliminate food in the intestines to keep your system running smoothly. Fiber also has properties that could help prevent gastro-intestinal ailments. A great source of fibrous complex carbohydrates is vegetables.

Besides giving the 'negative calorie effect' we discussed earlier, green veggies are filling, owing to their good fibrous content. Vegetables are also highly nutritious and not high in calories when compared to many processed foods. Nonetheless, some vegetables are superior especially when it comes to the negative calorie food list. The following are vegetables you should consider including in your diet.

Artichokes	Bean sprouts	Broccoli	Cabbage	Cauliflower
Asparagus	Beets and beet greens	Brussels sprouts	Carrots	Celery
Chives	Cucumbers	Green beans	Mushrooms	Peppers (red, green, yellow)
Pumpkin	Sauerkraut	Spinach	String beans	Turnips
Corn	Eggplant	Lettuce	Peas	Pickles
Radishes	Scallions	Squash	Tomatoes	Zucchini
Garlic	Onion	Watercress		

Fruits

Just like vegetables, fruits are a healthier option and always the recommended healthy alternative to sugary foods. It is therefore a better idea to snack on a bunch of grapes than it is to snack on candy.

However, when it comes to fruit choices, you also need to make better choices because some fruits are high in calories; thus, not providing you the negative calorie effect you are looking for in negative calorie foods

The list below contains some good negative-calorie fruits you can eat:

Apples	Blackberries	Cantaloupe	Cranberries	Grapefruit
Honeydew melon	Lemons	Mangoes	Apricots	Blueberries
Cherries	Currants	Grapes	Kiwi	Limes
Nectarines	Oranges	Pears	Pomegranates	Strawberries
Watermelon	Peaches	Pineapple	Raspberries	Tangerines
Prunes				

Herbs and spices

When it is a question of what you eat, even herbs and spices matter. Below is a complete list of herbs and spices you should always go for.

Chili pepper	Cloves	Ginger	Parsley	Cinnamon
Mustard seeds	Cayenne	Anise	Coriander/Cilantro	Dill
Cumin	Fennel seeds			

Meat, Fish and Seafood (Fats and Protein)

The whole idea behind negative calorie dieting revolves around weight loss; therefore, anything that supports this and still blends well with this kind of diet, a diet mainly comprised of vegetables and fruits can be considered. This is why we have to add a bit of fish, seafood, and meat to get fats and some protein.

Eating complex carbohydrates instead of simple carbohydrates is a great way to avoid gain weight, and having a method that reduces the possibility of taking simple carbohydrates is an even better way to avert the adverse effects of simple carbohydrates.

To explain this further, and the role of fats and some protein in all this, you first have to appreciate that we are eliminating all the bad carbohydrates (simple carbohydrates) and remaining with the good ones (complex carbohydrates).

The negative effect of simple carbohydrates

When you consume simple carbohydrates such as cakes, soda, juice, candy, white bread, pasta etc., your body easily converts them into glucose, which increases the blood sugar level rapidly.

This then triggers the release of insulin, which helps the sugar (glucose) get into your body cells for your body to use it as energy and the excess is converted into fat for storage. Thus, the main work of insulin is to assist you use the sugar you consume, or, if you are eating more than your body requires, store it as fat for later use.

Simple carbohydrates easily spike the insulin levels in your blood and the more you take them, the more you get fat (because the more fat your body stores). On the other hand, complex carbohydrates from fibrous foods take more time to digest and thus, apart from using up more calories to digest, they take a lot of time to increase insulin levels in your bloodstream.

Note: Your body requires energy, which it normally gets from carbohydrates. Having eliminated simple carbohydrates from your diet, it becomes harder for your body to get adequate energy; hence, it has to look for alternative sources of energy.

The role of fats (and changing the energy source)

When you begin consuming less carbohydrates and more fats, your body automatically begins burning fats to satisfy its energy requirements. In the process of burning fats, it produces molecules from the fats that the body then directly uses for energy. As your body adapts to the process of burning fats for energy, you gain from immense fat loss. Thus, this (incorporating fats), coupled with consuming complex, fibrous carbohydrates for the 'negative calorie effect', is an effective way to lose weight quickly.

The role of proteins

There are many ways through which proteins help you lose weight; the key ways include the following:

Important weight regulating hormones are changed

Your brain, and in particular, a section referred to as hypothalamus actively regulates your weight. To determine the time to eat and the amount of food to eat, your brain processes different types of information. Hormones are some of the most important signals to your brain and they change in response to eating.

When you take a high amount of protein, you increase the level of hormones that typically reduce appetite; these are cholecystokinin, GLP-1 and peptide YY. The hunger hormone, ghrelin, reduces in the process. The result is a significant drop in hunger, which is the major reason protein is helpful in weight loss.

Digestion and metabolizing proteins burns calories

When we eat , your body uses some of these calories to digest and metabolize the foods afterwards in a process we call the thermic effect of food, TEF. Even though we currently do not have sources that agree on the specific figures, it is rather clear that protein has a significant thermic effect: 20-30%. If you choose to go with a thermic effect of 30%, it means that 100 protein calories go down to 70 useful calories.

There are many other ways the right protein can enable help you to lose weight- but you get the idea.

Points to note when selecting the right proteins:

Red meat can be harmful to you, and many negative calorie diets don't recommend it; however, you do not have to avoid eating meat altogether, as it provides essential proteins and other nutrients. A good source of protein is fish for instance. Fish is lower in calories but high in essential nutrients like omega-3 fatty acids.

If you are allergic to fish, or if you are not a big fan of it, you can alternatively include small/reasonable potions of meat and chicken in your diet (I will teach you how in the recipes section).

The table below shows some of the best fish and seafood to include in your diet:

Clams	Crayfish	Mussels	Shrimp	Crab
Flounder	Tuna	Abalone	Buffalo fish	Cod
Terrapin	Bass	Catfish	Trout	

How To Make The Transition To Negative Calorie Diet

Now that you know what to eat, let us see exactly how you are going to be eating all that.

1. Make a smooth transition into the negative calorie diet so that you are comfortable with the entire process. Start by adding some negative calorie foods to the foods you normally eat in every meal in the 1:1 ratio. For instance, if having pasta with meatballs, you can serve 50% of this food and add chunks of zucchini to fill the other half.

You can also add a mixed salad to each meal you have; the salad should comprise of not less than 90% negative calorie foods. This means you have to look for ways to substitute any unwanted content such as any creamy high-fat substances with something like raspberry vinaigrette.

After some time, start slowly substituting the foods with the good (negative calorie) ones until your plate contains up to 90% negative calorie foods.

Note: We are only adding vegetables and fruits so far, not necessarily fully prepared negative calorie meals. Next, we will discuss the recipes so that you have entirely cooked meals too.

2. Use several vegetables to make a stir-fry. You can also make smoothie shakes with your favorite fruits including some berries. As said before, the negative calorie diet is largely a fruits and vegetables diet. However, this does not mean you should now start worrying about how you will survive as a vegetarian.

You can occasionally enjoy small servings of chicken and some meat, and the recipes in the following chapter will reflect that. Nonetheless, the meats have to be in small amounts; remember, you are losing weight and so, you have to make some sacrifices.

First Thing to Do

Buy all the foods you think you require from the list, wash, cut them into bits then seal them in airtight containers for storage (in the fridge) so that you will have them handy anytime you need them. You do not want to come home from work tired in the evening without having a bunch of these foods readily available. If you do, you will be extremely tempted to grab something unhealthy.

If you are wondering whether you will be hungry on this diet plan, just know that you will not because these foods are filling because they are high in fiber as well as water; the perfect combination to be full.

Note: While on this diet, you should have no room for alcohol, sugar, or any sugar substitutes except stevia simply because sugar intake causes your body to produce more insulin. This hormone signals/tells the fat cells to pick up and convert any excess glucose into fat. Therefore, eating more sugar means more production of insulin and consequently, more deposits in the fat cells. We are trying to reduce fat in your body, not create more of it. In this regard, avoid all commercial dressings since most of them contain sugar and high fat content.

Now that we have that out of the way, let us start cooking!

Negative Calorie Diet Recipes

While on a strict diet (such as this one), you might have a problem trying to decide what kind of dressing to use for your meals. Since I know it is important to be careful about what you are using, I will start by giving you two simple dressings that you will use on any meal you want.

Garlic and Herbs Dressing

Mix 1/2 cup of cold-pressed extra-virgin olive oil with juice from 1 lemon, 2 crushed garlic cloves and ¼ cup apple cider vinegar. Add some of your favorite negative calorie dried herbs such as parsley and cilantro.

This will yield 1 cup of dressing. Store the dressing in the fridge (for up to one month) to use on your foods.

Dijon and Yoghurt Dressing

For a delicious vegetable dip, mix Dijon mustard (2 tablespoons) with 2 cups low-fat yoghurt then add a pinch of chili pepper and a teaspoon of mixed dried herbs to spice it up.

Breakfast Recipes

Pumpkin Pancakes

Serves 4

Ingredients

1 cup of canned pumpkin

1 1/4 cups of water

2 teaspoons of cinnamon

2 cups Krusteaz pancake mix

1 egg, slightly beaten

1 teaspoon of baking powder

For the topping

1/4 cup of sliced pecans

5 tablespoons of pure maple syrup

Instructions

Combine all the ingredients for the pancake batter.

On a griddle or pan over medium heat sprayed with a little cooking spray, create a 10 cm circle of batter.

When the pancakes turn brown at the edges and you notice even bubbling across the top, flip them over to cook the other side.

In the meantime, toast pecans in a small pan until they turn slightly brown and give out the fragrance.

Serve with heated pure maple syrup.

Apple and Cinnamon with Almonds and Oat Bran

Serves 4

Ingredients

4 large apples

1 teaspoon of ground cinnamon

1/4 cup of oat bran

10 almonds, toasted and chopped

1 teaspoon of unrefined coconut oil

2 cups of unsweetened vanilla almond milk

2 packets monk fruit extract

Instructions

Wash the apples and cut into cubes.

Melt the coconut oil in a large nonstick skillet over medium high heat. Add the cinnamon and apples then cook for 2-3 minutes until the apples soften.

Remove from the heat, add almond milk, stir in the monk fruit extract and oat bran. Once mixed return back to the heat, stir, and bring to a simmer.

Cook for about one minute, until the mixture becomes thick and creamy.

Divide the mixture among four bowls then sprinkle each one with toasted almonds.

Negative Calorie Smoothie

Serves 2

Ingredients

5 strawberries

½ medium papaya

1 grapefruit

¼ cup ice

Instructions

Put all the ingredients in a blender; blend until smooth.

Serve and garnish with some strawberries and enjoy.

Berry Basil Smoothie

Servings 1

Ingredients

¾ cup almond milk

½ cup basil leaves

2 cups frozen strawberries

Instructions

Combine all the ingredients in a blender and process until smooth.

Lunch Recipes

Vegetable Soup

Serves 6

This is not your regular veggie soup; yes, it is simple, but it is full of negative calorie foods only.

Ingredients

6 cups of vegetable stock

1 cup of celery, diced

1 cup of green beans cut into about 1 inch pieces

1 medium zucchini, diced (approximately 2 cups)

1 cup small turnip, diced

1 jalapeno, seeded and finely chopped

1 medium onion, diced

1 cup of cauliflower florets

2 cups of shredded cabbage

3 cloves of garlic, finely chopped

2 cups of baby spinach

Salt and pepper to taste

Instructions

Mix the ingredients (except the spinach) in a pot, and bring to a boil.

Cover and let it simmer for 20 minutes.

Add the spinach, stir, and let it cook for one more minute.

Remove from the heat and serve.

Toast with Tomatoes

Serves 4

Ingredients

8 cups of spinach

½ ripe avocado, mashed well with a fork

Salt to taste

Freshly ground black pepper to taste

4 slices of natural gluten-free bread

4 (½-inch) slices ripe tomato

4 eggs, poached

Green hot sauce

Instructions

Place a nonstick skillet over medium high heat.

Add the spinach and cook until it wilts. Move the spinach to a colander and strain out as much water as possible. Put the now drained spinach in a bowl and season with green hot sauce and salt.

Use a toaster to toast the bread then season the avocado with salt. Evenly spread the pieces of avocado over each piece of toast then add a slice of tomato on top. Use pepper and salt to season the tomatoes and use the spinach mixture to top each slice evenly.

Place every piece of toast on a fresh plate. Finally, top with a poached egg and serve.

Meatballs with Mushroom Gravy

Serves 4

Ingredients

12 ounces lean ground beef

1 ounce Parmigiano Reggiano cheese, finely chopped

2 tablespoons arrowroot, dissolved in 2 teaspoons of stock

8 cups washed spinach

1 cup thinly sliced onion

4 cups sliced cremini mushrooms

Olive oil cooking spray

Freshly ground black pepper

Salt to taste

4 cups unsalted beef stock

1 cup finely chopped puffed brown rice

Instructions

Put the beef in a large bowl and push it to one side. Add rice and a cup of the stock to the other side of the mixing bowl; season with pepper and salt and allow the rice to absorb the stock for about 1 minute.

Mix the beef and rice using an electric hand mixture until well mixed. Taste and adjust the seasoning then use the mixture to form 16 meatballs.

Coat a skillet with olive oil cooking spray and place over medium heat. Once hot, put the meatballs and brown for one minute on one side. Turn and brown the opposite side for around 30 seconds and transfer to a plate.

Add the mushrooms to the skillet and sauté for a few minutes. Add the meatballs back to the skillet, then add the beef stock, arrowroot mixture, and cook until meatballs are cooked through.

Add the spinach and season with pepper and salt and cook until the spinach is wilted. Add the cheese, stir, and serve.

Chicken With Glazed Eggplant and Cauliflower Rice

Servings 4

Ingredients

1 tablespoon peeled and chopped fresh ginger

1 large clove garlic, thinly sliced

Red pepper flakes, to taste

1 ½ cups eggplant cut into 2-inch pieces

Kosher salt, to taste

3 tablespoons grated cauliflower

Olive oil cooking spray

4 ounces boneless, skinless chicken thighs scored crosswise 1/4 inch deep

1 tablespoon gluten-free reduced-sodium tamari

½ tablespoon balsamic vinegar

Instructions

Use cooking spray to spray a large nonstick pan and place the pan over medium high heat.

Add in the grated cauliflower and cook as you stir for a minute until just tender and softened.

Season with some red pepper flakes and salt then transfer to a plate and set aside.

Wipe the pan dry and spray again with cooking spray then place over medium heat.

Season the chicken with salt, add to pan to cook for about 2 minutes until brown on the outside, and done.

Transfer to a plate and set aside. Add the eggplant to the pan and cook for approximately 5 minutes until brown and soft.

Move the eggplant to one side of the pan and on the other side add garlic and cook for 30 seconds until browned.

Add ginger and cook for 15 more seconds until fragrant.

Add vinegar and tamari together with a splash of water and return the chicken back to the pan.

Cook for 30 seconds until the sauce coats everything and the chicken is cooked

Serve the chicken over rice and eggplant on the side.

Season with red pepper flakes and enjoy!

Dinner Recipes

Cabbage Soup

Serves 6

Ingredients

3 cups baby carrots

1 head cabbage

6 bouillon cubes

6 cups water

1 cup chopped celery

1 white onion

Instructions

Pour the water into a large saucepan, and then add the bouillon cubes into the water. Heat this over low heat.

Add the vegetables into the water, bring to a boil, increase heat to medium and cook until the vegetables are tender.

Brussels Sprouts with Lemon and Almond Dressing

Serves 3-4

Ingredients

3 pints Brussels sprouts, shaved thinly

5 teaspoons of freshly minced garlic

Crushed red pepper flakes

1/2 cup of chopped fresh flat-leaf parsley

Salt

1 1/2 teaspoons of extra-virgin olive oil

1/4 cup of toasted almonds, finely chopped

1/8 teaspoon of ground cinnamon

1/2 cup freshly squeezed lemon juice

1 ounce of Parmigiano-Reggiano cheese, finely grated

Instructions

Place the Brussels in a large mixing bowl and place it aside.

Place a non-stick skillet over medium high heat then add the garlic and olive oil. Cook until the garlic turns deep golden brown. Remove from the heat then add the parsley, almonds, cinnamon, and red pepper flakes.

Return the skillet back to the heat sauté for about ten seconds. Remove from the heat, pour in the lemon juice, and then season with salt.

Add the dressing to the Brussels then toss well, add 75% of the cheese, and toss some more. Taste then add the seasoning and top with the rest of the cheese.

Chicken with Pesto

Serves 3 or 4

Ingredients

Water

6 garlic cloves, chopped

Dash of paprika

1 cup of fresh basil leaves

8 cups of chopped escarole

Salt

1 ounce of Parmigiano-Reggiano cheese, finely grated

Olive oil cooking spray

Dash of cinnamon

Crushed red pepper flakes

1 small onion, thinly sliced

4 cups chicken stock, unsalted

12 ounces of skinless, boneless chicken breast sliced into 1/8 inch thick strips

Instructions

Pour 2 quarts of water in a medium pot and bring to a simmer. You will use this to poach the chicken.

Lightly coat a medium skillet with olive oil cooking spray then place it over medium high heat.

Add the garlic and cook until it turns golden brown. Add the cinnamon, basil leaves, red pepper flakes, onion, and paprika. Cook for roughly 2 minutes until the onion softens.

Add the escarole then cook until it is soft and wilted – for 2 more minutes. Add the stock, bring to a simmer, and then cover. Cook for about 5 minutes or until tender.

Add a pinch of salt to the simmering water and turn off the heat. Add the chicken and stir well until all parts separate. Cook until you notice the strips turning white (meaning they are half cooked). Use a slotted spoon to transfer the strips to a plate to cool.

Let the remaining mixture cook until most of the stock evaporates and looks like thick sauce or soup. Turn off the heat.

Add in half of the cheese, stir, and then season with salt to taste. Add the chicken strips then toss them to coat with the mixture and keep cooking until the strips have cooked enough through, for about 90 seconds.

Top with the remaining cheese, and then serve.

Vegetable Beef Soup

Serves 14

Note: This recipe has many ingredients and it is likely you will hate some vegetables or herbs. You can replace these vegetables and herbs with other ingredients on the negative calorie food list.

Ingredients

4 chopped onions

1 chopped red bell pepper

4 cups of sliced fresh mushrooms

10 chopped celery stalks with their leaves

2 cups of fresh chopped broccoli

1 small chopped bunch of cilantro

5 box low sodium beef broth

1 large chopped green bell pepper

4 cups of chopped cabbage

6 large chopped fresh carrots

1 finely chopped head of garlic

6 cups of fresh chopped spinach

1 small bunch of Parsley

1 can of asparagus (drained)

2 cans of green beans (drained)

1 cup of canned artichokes (drained)

20 twists of cracked black pepper

1 tablespoon of Italian seasoning

Protein (you can use just about any meat preferably the fishes mentioned in the list)

2 10 oz. cans of tomatoes with green chili's (not drained)

2 cans of diced tomatoes with basil (not drained)

1/2 tablespoon of red pepper flakes

1 tablespoon of dried basil

2 small cans of chopped green chilies (not drained)

1 lb. 80/20 or leaner ground beef (drain if needed)

Instructions

Fill a large cooking pot halfway with the beef, chicken, or vegetable stock. Add all the canned ingredients while draining some as specified into the pot.

Add water and all the spices then stir. Let it boil for some time, lower the heat to simmer for one hour or until the vegetables soften.

As the soup boils down, add some extra broth and stir.

Serve, garnish as desired, and enjoy.

Sea Bass with Spinach-Avocado Pesto

Servings 4

Ingredients

2 lemons, cut in half

Extra virgin olive oil

½ cup fresh parsley, chopped- plus more for garnish

Flaky sea salt

1 avocado, pitted

1 clove of garlic, smashed

¼ cup walnuts, chopped

2 teaspoons fresh lemon juice

4 pieces (about 2 pounds) wild Chilean sea bass

1 pound asparagus, ends trimmed

Freshly ground black pepper

2 cups baby spinach

Kosher salt

Instructions

Use pepper and salt to season the sea bass and set aside.

Add the parsley, walnuts, spinach, garlic and lemon juice, ¼ teaspoon pepper, ¼ cup olive oil and ½ teaspoon salt to the bowl of a food processor and pulse 2 to 3 times.

Add in the avocado and blend until well blended but the sauce still has some texture.

Place a large cast iron skillet over high heat. Add in a tablespoon of olive oil until almost smoking.

Add in the sea bass and sear it on all sides for 3 minutes each. Place on plate and set aside for 1 minute.

Return the iron skillet to medium high heat and add a teaspoon of olive oil, ½ teaspoon of salt and asparagus.

Brown for 5 minutes then transfer to a plate for serving.

Place the lemons, with the cut side down, in the skillet and adjust the heat to high. Sear the lemon for a minute.

Layer the sea bass on top of the asparagus then top with pesto and the seared lemon.

Garnish with parsley and sprinkle some sea salt on top.

Enjoy!

Chicken Meatballs with Quinoa & Curried Cauliflower

Servings 1

Ingredients

Handful dill, finely chopped

Pinch of cinnamon

1 garlic clove, finely chopped

2 spring onions, finely chopped

Pinch of cumin

250g chicken mince

1 teaspoon turmeric

For the quinoa and curried cauliflower:

1 tablespoon olive oil

½ lime- juiced

25g sweet potato, chopped

1 teaspoon sultanas

1 teaspoon pistachios, chopped

4 cauliflower florets

50g quinoa

1 tablespoon medium curry powder

Instructions

Mix all the meatball ingredients in a bowl together with some seasonings.

Use your hands to form six meatballs from the mixture then chill in the fridge for 20 minutes.

Preheat your oven to 200 degrees C/180 degrees C/ gas 6.

Wash the quinoa and add to a saucepan with 100 milliliters of water.

Bring to a boil then lower the heat to a gentle simmer and let it cook for about 10 to 15 minutes or until tender and doubled in size. Drain and set aside to cool.

Pour the sweet potato and cauliflower into a roasting tin and add in the curry powder and oil.

Place the meatballs in a different tin and cook both in the oven until cooked through, about 15 minutes.

Mix the quinoa with the sweet potato, sultanas, cauliflower, pistachios and squeeze the lime juice all over.

Serve this with the meatballs.

Snacks

Apple Chips

Serves 2

Ingredients

2 large granny smith apples

1 teaspoon of stevia

1 teaspoon of cinnamon

Canola oil cooking spray

Instructions

Preheat your oven to 200 degrees.

Using a sharp knife, thinly slice the apples crosswise. Arrange the slices on a single layer on a baking sheet then spray with canola oil cooking spray.

Evenly sprinkle the stevia and cinnamon over the apple slices.

Use the bottom third part of the oven to bake the apples until they are crisp and dry, roughly 2-2½ hours.

Alternatively, you could use a mastrad chipmaker. Not only is it easy and fast, you do not need the cooking spray. Just lay the apple slices on the chipmaker, sprinkle with cinnamon and stevia, and then microwave for 4-5 minutes.

Berry Salad

Serves 4

Ingredients

4 cups of mixed berries (blackberries, raspberries, blueberries, strawberries)

20 whole almonds, toasted and chopped

2 tablespoons of hemp hearts

1/4 cup of cooked quinoa

1 ½ tablespoons of fat free yoghurt

Instructions

Divide all the ingredients equally among four bowls and toss well to mix.

Fruit Salad

Serves 10

Ingredients

2/3 cup of fresh orange juice

1/2 teaspoon of grated lemon zest

2 cups of cubed fresh pineapple

3 kiwi fruits, peeled and sliced

2 oranges, peeled and sectioned

2 cups of blueberries

1/3 cup of fresh lemon juice

1/2 teaspoon of grated orange zest

1 teaspoon of vanilla extract

2 cups of strawberries, hulled and sliced

3 bananas, sliced

1 cup seedless grapes

Instructions

Add orange zest, orange juice, lemon juice and lemon zest, to a saucepan, place it over medium high heat, and bring to boil.

Decrease the heat to medium-low and let it simmer for 5 minutes. Remove from the heat and stir in the vanilla extract. Place it aside to cool.

Place the fruit in a clear glass bowl in layers starting with the pineapple, then strawberries, kiwi, bananas, oranges, then grapes and at the top, blueberries.

Pour the juice over the fruit layers then cover and leave in the fridge for 3-4 hours before serving.

Almond Cake with Berries

Serves 4

Ingredients

½ cup of almond meal

4 packets of monk fruit extract

1 teaspoon of vanilla extract

Olive oil cooking spray

2 eggs, separated; remove 1 yolk

3 tablespoons of raw coconut nectar

Salt

1 cup of mixed berries, mashed well with a fork

Instructions

Preheat your oven to 3750 degrees F.

Bake the almond meal until it becomes aromatic and well toasted –about 3-5 minutes. Remove from the oven and place it on a cool baking sheet.

Place the monk fruit and egg whites in a bowl and whisk until it forms stiff peaks. Use cooking spray to spray four paper cups. Using a toothpick or fork, poke holes in the bottom of each.

Place the almond meal into a mixing bowl then add the egg yolk, salt, vanilla, and coconut nectar. Fold the meringue into the mixture of almond and transfer the batter into the cups.

Place in the microwave and microwave for about thirty seconds. When the mixture has cooked through, place the cups on their sides and give them 45 seconds to cook.

Remove the cakes and place them upside down on four serving plates.

Get them off the cups and serve with berries.

Cucumber and salsa

Serves 2

Ingredients

2 cucumbers, peeled and sliced

12 garlic cloves, minced

¼ cup fresh cilantro, chopped

3 tomatoes, diced

½ sweet onion, diced

Sea salt and black pepper to taste

Instructions

Mix all ingredients except the cucumber in a bowl in order to make the salsa.

Place cucumber slices on a plate and serve with the salsa.

Pineapple and Berry Hemp Seed Pudding

Servings 3

Ingredients

2 tablespoons hemp seeds

1 cup pineapple, cubed

2 cups organic berries (fresh or, if frozen, thawed)

2 tablespoons chia seeds

2 tablespoons light coconut milk (or almond milk)

1/8 teaspoon ground cinnamon

Optional: maple syrup or pitted dates to taste

Instructions

Place the coconut milk, pineappe and berries into a food processor and mix until combined.

Taste and adjust the sweetness as desired with either pitted dates or maple syrup (optional) and then blend to combine.

Now add the cinnamon, hemp seeds and chia seeds and pulse until nicely combined.

Transfer the mixture to 3 to 4 serving dishes, cover and refrigerate for about 2 hours to chill (or overnight).

You can keep this in the refrigerator for up to 3 to 4 days.

Notes

For the berries, you can use a mixture of strawberries, raspberries, blackberries or other berries of choice.

You can use 1 to 2 tablespoons of chia seeds or flaxseed meal if you have trouble digesting chia seeds.

Kale and Berry Smoothie

Servings 2

Ingredients

1 teaspoon ground flaxseed

1 apple, cored and cut into pieces

1 cup frozen organic berries

½ cup (packed) flat-leaf parsley (leaves and stems)

4 kale leaves (center ribs removed)

Instructions

Toss all the ingredients together with 1 cup of water into your blender and puree until smooth. If the smoothie is too thick, thin it with a bit more water.

Pour into 2 glasses and enjoy!

Negative Calorie Diet And Exercise: An Effective Way To Lose Weight Fast

I promised you some unique and cool exercise tips, right? Doing the following exercises will help you burn the fat much faster. All you have to do is to start slow and over time, increase the intensity, keep an open mind, and use the gym (for the ones that require it), where you have an instructor nearby.

Interval Training

This is all about high intensity exercises combined with short periods of rest. This will not only burn more calories than your typical cardio training, it will boost your body's ability to burn fat easily since it increases the production of the growth hormone, which is also a fat burning hormone, and adrenaline which assists in suppressing your appetite.

The intervals will work on your muscles, and help them use oxygen better so that your heart does not have to struggle to pump a lot to make them perform.

Do It!

Get on a treadmill or a stationary bike then use the guide below to start your own interval-training regimen:

Begin with a regular warm-up (any simple exercise to get your blood rushing). When done, run or pedal at a rate that is more than your regular cardio intensity by 20%. If you have never engaged in any serious cardio workouts before, you might want to check this first to understand what I am talking about.

After 30 seconds to 1 minute, reduce the intensity to a rate that is 50% less than the intensity of a regular cardio workout. Alternate the periods of 30 seconds to 1 minute of hard work with 30 seconds to 1 minute of relaxed pedaling or if you want, relaxed running for 6-10 intervals to finish your session.

As this gets simpler, increase each interval's intensity so that you work even longer during the difficult part, reduce your rest periods, or if you feel enthusiastic enough, add more intervals.

Repeat 3-4 times each week.

As you get the hang of this exercise, start the next:

Sprinting

Try sprinting up a hill since the impact on your joints will be much lower and can help you avoid injury. If there is no hilly ground in your area, try the alternative: the dag race approach. Start your sprint by increasing your speed from a jog.

To make the most of this exercise, keep the sprints short – ideally 50 yards per sprint. This helps you sustain a high intensity all through and prevents injury.

If you want to increase the overall results of your sprint workout, increase your total number of sprints. This is better than going for long distance runs.

If you are new to exercising, do not do more than one workout per week. You can increase the days once you accustom to the exercise; just remember to allow at least two days of recovery between the workouts.

High Intensity Strength Intervals

Select two exercises that work different muscles completely or ones that use opposite movements. For instance, you can pair a pulling exercise with a pushing exercise or upper body exercise with a lower body exercise like pull-ups and squats.

For the latter, select a weight (if your instructor thinks you need one) with which you can do 10 repetitions. Alternate between the two exercises and do just five repetitions of each move in every set. Remember to rest between the sets so that you finish each set without failing.

Keep alternating between the exercises for a 10 or 15 minutes set time. Keep noting the total number of sets you can do. In subsequent sessions, try to beat your score by completing more sets in the same duration or completing the same number of sets but with heavier weights.

As you get the hang of the above exercises, start the next:

Countdown Workouts

Countdown workouts fit in the use of exercise pairs really well. They also keep you fully engaged in the exercises since you have to keep the count and pay attention.

With every round of the exercise pair, the training encompasses one lesser rep of each move; for instance, you move from a set of six to five...until zero.

You can also try density training where you pair opposing exercises for countdowns. For instance, kettlebell swing, pushups, and squat thrusts would work really well.

Do it!

Start by selecting your pair of exercises.

Perform six repetitions of the first exercise, then six reps of the other move. Go back to the first move and perform five reps then five more of the second exercise. Keep alternating until you reach zero.

In the subsequent workouts, add one rep to each exercise. If you want more countdowns, select a second pair from the list below, or just come up with your own pair of opposing moves.

Squat thrust, pushups

Kettlebell swing, squat thrust

Jumping jacks, pushups

Medicine ball side toss, medicine ball slam

As you get the hang of the above exercise, start the next:

Hurricane Workouts

This is essentially a workout protocol that entails lifting weights and interval training. We have three groups of exercises, called rounds in this type of workouts. Each round has an exercise that increases your heart rate, and a set of other exercises in between.

This design will allow you to keep your heart rate up throughout the workout (and burn significant amounts of calories) that typically lasts 16-22 minutes. Hurricane workouts have five levels and each one is an increased challenge. I have however prepared for you a sample routine you will work with below.

Note: This will require you to be more fit- if fit enough though, you can begin with this:

Warm up for the workout. For all rounds, do one set of each exercise and move on to the next exercise. Finish the whole round thrice before you move to the next round.

First round: Run on a treadmill at 10% incline, 10.5 mph for 25 seconds. Do a kettlebell Turkish get up about 4 times on each side of your body then 10 chin-ups.

Repeat this sequence thrice.

Second round: Run on a treadmill at a 10% incline, 11 mph for 25 seconds. Do 10 dips and a barbell rollout, 15 reps.

Repeat this process thrice.

Third round: Run on a treadmill at a 10% incline, 11.5 mph for 25 seconds. Perform the G.I row, 10 reps. Do the knee grab, 20 reps.

Repeat three times.

Final Note

Remember, obesity is a condition linked to a higher risk of cardiovascular disease, type II diabetes, psychological illnesses and many other conditions and diseases. Losing weight can decrease the risks of these and other issues associated with obesity, and decrease the severity of the symptoms if you already have the diseases. Trying this diet is worth all your effort.

Apart from the illnesses, you also have to consider the ultimate purpose of living for most of us, and this is attaining happiness and inner peace. Losing excess weight, even a single pound of it, brings some level of happiness to most of us. In fact, you do not necessarily have to attain your goal weight in order to be happy. For instance, there was a study conducted in 2009 on 900 weight loss patients. From this group, those who managed to reduce 5-10% of their total body weight had better scores on measures of self-esteem and physical function.

Just being aware that losing weight helps a lot in these areas is another good way to keep yourself motivated to lose more, even when you feel like quitting exercising or the negative calorie diet.

I need your help...

Thank you for buying this book!

I hope this book was able to help you to know more about the Negative Calorie Diet and how you can burn fat and lose weight with this diet, the next step is to put what you have learned into practice and actually adopt the diet if you want to see those pounds coming off.

Finally, if you enjoyed this book, would you be kind enough to leave a review for this book on Amazon?

Please leave a review for this book on Amazon!

I want to reach as many people as I can with this book, and more reviews will help me accomplish that!

If you have any questions or problems, please contact us: hello@freedomdestination.com

Thank you and good luck!

Preview Of 'Belly Diet'

You've heard and read much about the Zero Belly diet. But it's possible that you've heard and read wrong, given that the Zero Belly diet is like a Hollywood celebrity who's subject to lots of news and speculations, some of them true and a lot of them not. So really, what's the diet all about?

Essentially, the Zero Belly diet is – as the name suggests – an eating plan that can help you achieve a significantly tighter waistline (zero or near zero belly) and in the process, burn much body fat in as little as 2 weeks – or less. The Zero Belly diet was conceptualized by a diet professional by the name of David Zinczenko. If his name sounds kind of familiar, blame it on the fact that he's the author of one of the most popular diet books Eat This, Not That – popular enough to land on the New York Times Bestseller list. And if you're still not convinced of who the dude is, check this out – he was the former editor-in-chief of one of the most health and fitness conscious magazines in the world called Men's Health.

The diet's main USP or unique selling proposition is the claim to provide you with a new and revolutionary eating plan that will help you lose significant body fat in quite a short time and keep it off for life. Even more interesting – and intriguing, if I may add – is the claim that you can achieve a flat or substantially flatter belly in that short amount of time with 3 big No's – no exercising, no dieting, and no worrying. I can hear a choir of angels singing right now...hallelujah! I know, right?

I can hear your skeptical mind thinking aloud: "Really? It's that quick and easy? How does it work?" I hear ya!

The Zero Belly Diet General Protocols

In order for you to achieve the diet's promises, there are several things you'll need to strictly observe, with the exception of one optional item. These are:

- You can maximize the amount of body fat you can lose by undergoing an optional cleanse for 7 days, just before you begin the actual Zero Belly Diet process. This will involve eating restrictions in order to help prime up your body for the Zero Belly phase. It can also help you kick start your fat loss by helping you lose some pounds too.

- For the most part, you will need to eat foods that are plant-based. Take note, I wrote "most part", which means meat and fish aren't illegal but merely limited in quantity. However, you can enjoy eggs in the morning as you kick-start your day with breakfast.

- Most of the food you'll eat will involve fruits, veggies, healthy fats, seeds, nuts, legumes, and lean sources of protein.

- Minimize or avoid altogether your consumption of processed foods, sugar, dairy products, refined grains, and glutinous foods.

The Purge, I Mean The (Optional) Cleanse

As mentioned earlier, the diet features an optional 7-day cleanse prior to proceeding to the main diet itself, which is a great way to kick start and optimize your fat burning efforts under the Zero Belly diet. You can also use this cleanse apart from the diet itself to detoxify your body after a party-everyday-till-you-drop kind of summer vacation.

So how do you do the 7-day cleanse? Here's how:

- Your daily cleanse will be made up of having a Zero Belly drink for your breakfast, another one during lunch, a snack at any point within the day, and one Zero Belly cleansing dinner. Sorry, no desserts allowed in this phase.

- There must be protein, healthy fats, and dietary fiber in everything you consume during the cleansing week, i.e., your meals, snacks, and drinks.

- For your cleansing dinners, these must be made of healthy fats, veggies, and lean protein. Fruits and grains are banned during the 7-day cleanse.

- The 7-day purge is really that – a purge – as it bans cheat meals and alcoholic drinks for the cleanse's duration.

- Your daily water consumption should be no less than 8 glasses.

- If you'd like to maximize your fat loss, another good option is to drink up 3 to 4 cups of white, red, rooibos, oolong, mint, and green teas daily.

The Zero Belly Rules

While the enjoyable features of the Zero Belly diet are made up of the word "No", it doesn't mean it's total anarchy as far as your eating is concerned. As a diet, it still has several rules that you'll need to abide by in order to experience substantial fat loss and achieve a flat (or significantly flatter belly) in just 2 weeks. These rules include:

- Three Squared: You'll need to eat 3 square meals every day. No more, no less.

- You can drink a maximum of 1 serving of any Zero Belly drink daily.

- If you're still hungry in between your meals, you're allowed to munch one snack in the afternoon or evening.

- When you're eating, don't do anything else, e.g., don't watch TV, read the papers, or engage in a conversation. Why? It's because when you eat mindlessly or with distractions, you'll tend to eat more than what's enough to make you feel reasonably full. If you eat that way, how can you lose body fat in any diet?

- You can enjoy one meal of your food of choice, i.e., cheat meal, every week.

- You can have a cup of your favorite coffee daily and an alcoholic drink every week.

Allowed

Earlier in the discussion on general protocols, I gave you a general idea of the best foods to eat in the Zero Belly diet. Here's a more specific list of the foods that are allowed during your Zero Belly diet period:

Phyto-Nutritious Veggies

Veggies that have a lot of green leaves or are brightly colored such as asparagus, arugula, beets, avocados, bell peppers, beet greens, chard, carrots, collard greens, chicory, lettuce, kale, spinach, parsley, turnips, zucchini, and tomatoes. You may also include sweet potatoes, peas, scallions, mushrooms, leeks, onions, and garlic in your daily menu.

Phyto-Nutritious Fruits

If you're the type who loves to eat fruits – rejoice! Unlike other fat loss diets, you can eat fruits in the Zero Belly diet. The diet prioritizes red-colored fruits like tart cherries, apples, grapefruits, grapes, strawberries, watermelon and raspberries. If you find it hard to get your fix of red-colored fruits, you can eat plums, peaches, and blueberries instead.

Low Or Non-Fat Proteins

When it comes to proteins, the Zero Belly diet is generally accommodating to lean cuts of the stuff. In fact, the diet encourages the consumption of lean protein sources such as oysters, organic eggs, shrimps, scallops, chicken and turkey breasts, cod, anchovies, halibut, tuna, trout, sardines, tuna, and white fish. Vegan or plant-based protein powders or shakes are also accepted in the Zero Belly diet, with each scoop containing at least 15 grams of protein per scoop. Whey protein – unfortunately – is a dairy-based protein source and as such, is discouraged in the Zero Belly diet.

Good Fats

Yes – there is such a thing as good fat. These are the monounsaturated fats that are mostly available in olives and their derivative oils, seeds, nuts, dark chocolates (at least 72% cacao and very little or no sugar), avocados. Polyunsaturated fats are also considered good fats and are generally available from oily fishes such as sardines, mackerel, salmon and tuna. Polyunsaturated fat can also come from flaxseeds, pine nuts, sesame seeds, and sunflower seeds. Other less preferred – but still allowed nonetheless – sources of healthy fats include coconuts and their derivative oils (coconut oil), grass-fed cows, fish that thrive in cold water, chia seeds, and walnuts.

Nuts And Seeds

Given that you are allowed to eat nuts and seeds in the Zero Belly diet, it's important that you know what and how to eat them. If you love eating nuts such as cashews, almonds, hazelnuts, coconuts, pine nuts, peanuts, and walnuts, you should eat them raw and without any salt. The same goes for seeds like pumpkin, ground flax, and chia seeds. If you like to eat almond or peanut butter, that's alright under the Zero Belly diet for as long as you're certain that such butters are made mostly – if not entirely – of the seed or the nut with just a bit of salt.

Flavorings

To add more zest and spice to your Zero Belly meals, you can use certain types of flavorings such as herbs, spices, and condiments. For herbs and spices, you're practically free to flavor your food with the most popular, ones like black pepper (whole or ground), paprika, curry, and oregano, among others. If you're the type who enjoys adding some chocolate to enhance the flavor of food, you can use dark chocolates too, as long as it's at least 70% cocoa, as mentioned earlier.

When it comes to condiments, the Zero Belly diet's a bit strict about it in that you have limited options to choose from. Nevertheless, the allowed condiments in the Zero Belly diet can add a lot of flavor to your dishes. These include rice wine vinegar, apple cider vinegar, white wine vinegar, red wine vinegar, red curry paste, prepared mustard, Sriracha sauce, low sodium soy sauce, and organic salsa.

Diet Drinks

No, we ain't talkin' about sugar-free versions of your favorite soda or iced tea here. We're talking about drinks that are encouraged, required actually, in the diet. These include plain drinking water, unsweetened almond milk, hazelnut milk, coconut milk, oat milk, rice milk, and green tea. Only dairy milk is banned from the diet because it comes from cows. Seriously, it's because dairy-based products are banned from the Zero Belly diet.

As for water consumption, drink a glass first thing in the morning, a glass each with every meal, and in between meals to get at least 8 glasses everyday. Other deliciously satisfying Zero Belly approved diet drinks include smoothies made from fruits, veggies, and the above-mentioned milk.

Others

You can also consume grains and legumes when on the Zero Belly diet. For grains, just stick to brown rice, barley, oats, quinoa, and rye. If you're going to eat a sandwich, make sure that the bread or bun you'll eat are gluten-free. For legumes, you can eat peanuts, chickpeas, kidney beans, black beans, lentils, and pinto beans.

Not Allowed

Of course, any diet wouldn't be such without limiting or banning certain types of food. Apart from dairy-based products, the following are foods that you either need to limit or eliminate altogether.

Limited Consumption

- Alcoholic beverages

- Coffee

- Flatulence-causing veggies such as cauliflower, cabbage, Brussels sprouts, and broccoli

- Omega 6 Fatty Acids that are abundant in foods such as sunflower seeds, mayonnaise, grape seed oil, cottonseed oil, sesame oil, vegetable oil, poppy seed oil, and soybean oil

- Red meat and proteins in general;

- Soy milk

- Sweetening agents like brown sugar and honey

Banned

- Canned foods

- Dairy products, including yogurt

- Fruit juices

- Low phytonutrient content foods like white root vegetables (parsnips and turnips)

- Processed foods

- Refined grains

- Saturated fats

- Soy protein, sorbitol, fructose, salty foods, carrageenan, and other flatulence-inducing foods

- Sugar

- Wheat

Exercise

While the Zero Belly diet doesn't require you to exercise to achieve a flat or substantially flatter belly in just 2 weeks, adding it to the diet will help you maximize the – pardon the pun – flat belly fits of the diet by helping you burn more fat than if you merely dieted alone. So if you'd like to really crank up your fat loss during the 2-week period, exercising is highly recommended.

What types of exercises should you do? Nothing fancy really. You don't need to do grueling exercise routines. Simple exercises such as brisk walking, running, and easy bodyweight exercises such as squats or modified pushups can do wonders in conjunction with the Zero Belly diet.

The key here is to perform exercises that involve several muscles for at least 30 straight minutes at moderate intensity. The exercises I mentioned above use several muscles at a time. For example, squats involve the use of your thighs, butt, leg, and core muscles. The more muscles are involved in a particular exercise, the more calories are burned.

To measure the intensity of your exercise, use the talk test. Exercise for 2 to 3 minutes straight and try to talk. If you're able to talk normally without any effort, it's too easy – light intensity. If you're panting and are barely able to talk, that's too hard – high intensity. If you're able to carry a conversation with a little effort, that's just right – moderate intensity.

Zero Belly Benefits

Apart from flattening your tummy, there are other benefits that can be associated with the diet. Generally speaking, fat loss can help bring down your risks for major diseases. In specific terms, Zinczenko claims the diet he created can help lower risks for the following:

- Anxiety

- Alzheimer's Disease

- Autoimmune Diseases

- Arthritis

- Bloating

- Barrett's Esophagus

- Dementia

- Certain Types Of Cancer

- Depression

- Flatulence (hey, that's an embarrassing social condition)

- Diabetes

- Heart Disease

- Gastro-Esophageal Reflux Disease or GERD

- Inflammation

- High Blood Sugar

- Low Sex Drive

- Liver Disease

- Obesity

- Memory Loss

- Visceral Fat

- Stroke

- Psoriasis

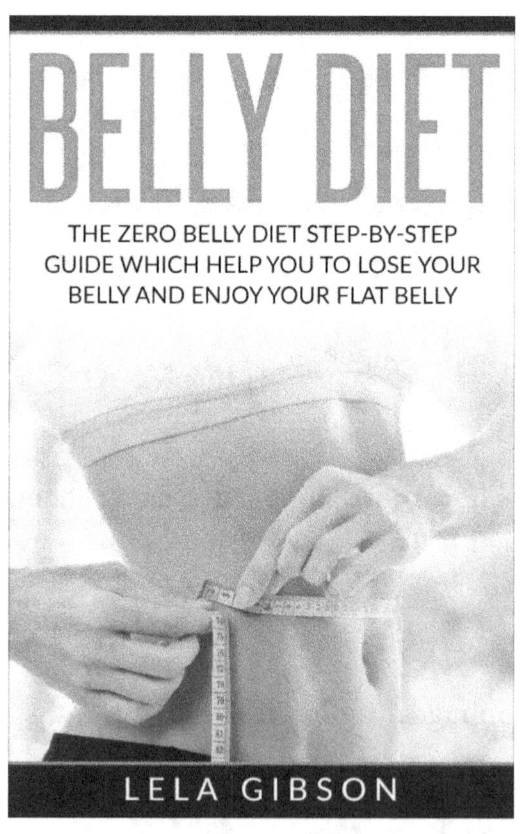

Check out the rest of The Belly Diet on Amazon.here: http://bit.ly/belly-diet

Check Out My Other Books

Below you'll find some of my other popular books that are popular on Amazon and Kindle as well.

Alternatively, you can visit my author page on Amazon to see other work done by me.

20 Easy And Fast Diet Tips For Losing Weight – An Easy-To-Follow Weight Loss Guide

Belly Diet: The Zero Belly Diet Step-By-Step Guide Which Will Help You To Lose Your Belly And Enjoy Your Flat Belly

Anti-Inflammatory Diet Guide – The Guide To Reduce Inflammation And Live A Healthy Life Without Pain

Dash Diet: Cookbook For Weight Loss With Action Plan And Easy Recipes

Clean Eating: Cookbook And Guide To Restore Your Body's Natural Balance And Eat Healthy

<u>Negative Calorie Diet: Cookbook & Guide Which Help You To Burn Body Fat, Lose Weight And Live Healthy</u>

<u>Smart Fat: Cookbook With Fat Meals Which Help You To Lose Weight, Get Healthy And Improve Brain Function</u>

www.ingramcontent.com/pod-product-compliance
Lightning Source LLC
Chambersburg PA
CBHW070032260726
48658CB00002B/595